The Fundamental Role of the Arts and Humanities in Medical Education

Lisa Howley, PhD
Elizabeth Gaufberg, MD, MPH
Brandy King, MLIS

Association of American Medical Colleges
Washington, D.C.

The report was funded, in part, by the Josiah Macy Jr. Foundation. Any views, findings, conclusions, or recommendations expressed here and in related programming or products do not represent those of the foundation or any other grantors.

The AAMC (Association of American Medical Colleges) is a not-for-profit association dedicated to transforming health through medical education, health care, medical research, and community collaborations. Its members are all 155 accredited U.S. and 17 accredited Canadian medical schools; more than 400 teaching hospitals and health systems, including Department of Veterans Affairs medical centers; and more than 70 academic societies. Through these institutions and organizations, the AAMC leads and serves America's medical schools and teaching hospitals and their more than 179,000 full-time faculty members, 92,000 medical students, 140,000 resident physicians, and 60,000 graduate students and postdoctoral researchers in the biomedical sciences. Additional information about the AAMC is available at aamc.org.

ISBN: 978-1-57754-194-3

Suggested citation: Howley L, Gaufberg E, King B. *The Fundamental Role of the Arts and Humanities in Medical Education.* Washington, DC: AAMC; 2020.

AAMC

Contents

Acknowledgments *v*

Executive Summary *1*

1. Purpose of the Report *3*

2. Introduction and Historical Context *5*
What do we mean by the integration of arts and humanities in medicine? *5*
How did we get here? *6*

3. The Fundamental Role of the Arts and Humanities in Medical Education and Physician Development *9*
How are the arts and humanities integrated within medical education? *9*
What role do these approaches play in competency-based education? *10*
What are barriers to integration? *10*
What are key functions of integrative curricula? *10*
What are some examples of using arts and humanities interventions to foster teamwork and collaboration, resilience, and flexibility? *12*
What are deliberate pedagogies for integrative curricula? *13*
What are effective methods for study and evaluation? *14*

4. Current Landscape and Research Needs *17*
What is the scope of published literature on arts and humanities in medical education? *17*
What are research gaps and areas for future study? *18*
What factors support the growth of arts and humanities integration? *19*

5. Examples of Integrative Approaches *21*
Training the Eye by Joel Katz, MD (Visual Arts) *22*
Narrative Medicine by Rita Charon, MD, PhD (Narrative Medicine) *22*
The Art of Communication by Karen Novak, DDS, PhD (Visual Arts) *22*
Playing Doctor by Katie Watson, JD (Theater and Drama) *23*
My Life, My Story by Susan Nathan, MD (Reflective Writing) *24*
Medical Readers' Theater by Todd Savitt, PhD, and Sheena Eagan, MPH, PhD (Theater and Drama) *24*
Jazz and the Art of Medicine by Paul Haidet, MD (Music) *24*
Literature and Medicine by Dan Marchalik, MD (Literature) *25*
History of Medicine by Jeremy Greene, MD, PhD (History) *25*
Documentary Film by Maren Monsen, MD (Film and Television) *25*
Dance for All People by Rachel Balaban (Dance and Movement) *26*
The College Colloquium by Quentin Eichbaum, MD, PhD, MPH, MFA (Mixed) *26*
The Art of Medicine by Allison Bickett, PhD, and Mary Hall, MD (Visual Arts) *27*

6. Recommendations for Integrative Approaches *29*

Conclusions *31*

Appendix A. FRAHME Methods and Strategy *33*

Appendix B. FRAHME Roster *35*

References *39*

AAMC

Acknowledgments

The AAMC acknowledges the dedication and support of the many individuals, teams, and organizations that contributed to the development of this report.

The Josiah Macy Jr. Foundation provided grant funding (P19-02) to support the report's development, and the National Endowment for the Humanities (NEH) has provided funding (AH-268665-19) to support a broader initiative, the Fundamental Role of the Arts and Humanities in Medical Education (FRAHME): A National Strategic Initiative to Further Advance Curricular Integration of the Humanities and Arts into U.S. Medical Schools and Teaching Hospitals. We deeply appreciate the Josiah Macy Jr. Foundation and the NEH for supporting this work. We also extend our gratitude to Gerald Lazarus, MD, and the Board of the National Trust for the Humanities.

The Scoping Review Team, commissioned in 2019, provided a rich understanding of the current landscape of the published literature in this educational area and areas for further exploration. We thank them for their efforts to advance our collective understanding of the science behind these integrative practices. The members of the FRAHME Integration Committee guided and shaped the concepts in this report, and we extend our deep appreciation and regard for their efforts and expertise. Names of the members of the Scoping Review Team and the Integration Committee can be found in Appendix B.

We also extend our appreciation to Virginia Bush, PMP, AAMC project manager, and the talented AAMC Communications team, including Cindy Allen, Caren Clark, Mukti Desai, Mark Mavilia, and Lindsay Tiffany, for their efforts toward the production of this report. We recognize the collaborative support, executive sponsorship, and leadership of Alison Whelan, MD, AAMC chief medical education officer. We also thank David Skorton, MD, AAMC president, and Darrell Kirch, MD, AAMC president emeritus, for their enduring vision and commitment to integrating the arts and humanities into medical education to improve clinician well-being and better patient care for all.

Lisa Howley, PhD, AAMC Senior Director of Strategic Initiatives and Partnerships in Medical Education

Elizabeth Gaufberg, MD, MPH, AAMC Senior Consultant, Associate Professor of Medicine and Psychiatry, Harvard Medical School

Brandy King, MLIS, FSLA, AAMC Senior Consultant

Executive Summary

The first two decades of 21st-century medicine have witnessed significant transformation in health care delivery, marked health disparities, civil unrest, unprecedented rates of physician burnout and suicide, and unforeseen public health crises in the forms of the opioid epidemic and the coronavirus pandemic. Physicians must be adaptive lifelong learners who can effectively respond to these and future challenges. Now more than ever, physicians must learn to interweave their developing scientific knowledge with emotional intelligence, critical thinking skills, and an understanding of social context. The integration of the arts and humanities into medicine and medical education may be essential to educating a physician workforce that can effectively contribute to optimal health care outcomes for patients and communities.

The AAMC believes the arts and the humanities can play a unique and unrealized role in preparing and equipping physicians for 21st-century challenges. Specifically, we propose the following recommendations for the academic medicine community:

1. Assert that the practice of medicine is an art as well as a science, requiring a grounding in humanistic values, principles, and skills, including a deep understanding of the human condition.

2. Create more effective arts and humanities integrative models for competency-based teaching and learning in medicine.

3. Enhance the research and evaluation of courses and programs that integrate the arts and humanities into medical education and continuing professional development. Such research and evaluation should include measuring learner outcomes beyond satisfaction with the course or program and should follow sound scholarly practices.

4. Design approaches to enhancing trainee and physician well-being that integrate the arts and humanities into medicine.

5. Increase collaboration among scholars of higher education, medical professionals, arts organizations, creative arts therapists, artists, humanities scholars, learners, and patients.

6. Provide professional development offerings that enhance faculties' capacity to design curricula and facilitate the use of models that integrate the arts, humanities, and medicine in training.

7. Investigate effective integrative pedagogical practices and recognize an expansive view of scholarship in academic promotion and tenure processes.

The AAMC FRAHME (Fundamental Role of the Arts and Humanities in Medical Education) initiative advances arts and humanities integration into medical education to improve the education, practice, and well-being of physicians and physician learners across the continuum. New strategies, research, and scholarship in integrative arts and humanities curricula abound, but the content, pedagogy, degree of integration, effective assessment, and evaluation methods vary.

This report reviews the historic and current state of arts and humanities integration into medical education, considers curriculum and assessment methods, and provides guidance on the research and change in culture necessary for effective integration. We present the findings of a commissioned scoping review of the literature on arts and humanities integration and an emerging theory of practice, the Prism Model, to support arts and humanities curriculum development. We review factors supporting the growth of arts and humanities integration and strategies to overcome barriers, and we feature example programs — including narrative medicine, improvisation, visual arts, music, theater arts, and the study of history — designed to achieve important learning outcomes.

Recommendations for the future of this foundational field include tighter linkage of educational offerings to core competencies, enhancement of research and evaluation methods, more opportunities for professional development, and greater collaboration among faculty, learners, patients, and arts and humanities partners in the process of curriculum design. We offer this report to inform dialogue and guide action in harnessing the multifaceted role the arts and humanities may play in transforming medical education to meet 21st-century health care needs and our broader quadruple aim to enhance the patient experience, improve population health, reduce costs, and promote clinician well-being.

Wherever the art of Medicine is loved, there is also a love of Humanity. — Hippocrates

1. Purpose of the Report

The AAMC is dedicated to articulating the critical foundations for the education of future physicians, as well as new competencies and pedagogical practices for teaching and learning across the medical education continuum. The time is right to define the role the arts and humanities play in the initial and ongoing development of physicians. In 2009, the AAMC, in collaboration with the Howard Hughes Medical Institute, published the first of its Foundations monographs, *The Scientific Foundations for Future Physicians.*[1] The AAMC published the second Foundations monograph, *Behavioral and Social Science Foundations for Future Physicians*, in 2011.[2] These Foundations documents, distributed widely to medical educators, guide curricular planning and execution.

In 2017, the AAMC decided a third monograph was needed to provide a more complete picture of the the essential foundations for educating physicians. Unlike the earlier two monographs, which address the development of physicians in medical school, this one also addresses the development of physicians in residency and in practice. This work is part of a broader AAMC strategic initiative, the Fundamental Role of the Arts and Humanities in Medical Education (FRAHME). The primary goal of this longitudinal, cross-continuum initiative is to **improve the education, practice, and well-being of physicians through deeper integrative experiences with the arts and humanities**. Included in this broader initiative are the design and launch of a digital guidebook with practical tools for integrating arts and humanities into medical education curricula and experiences.

Similar to the earlier two monographs, this one is not intended as a mandate for curricular or program reform. Instead, it is a guide to help medical educators and practicing clinicians understand the value of further integrating the arts and humanities into their teaching and learning practices. We identify competencies and outcomes that arts-and-humanities-based pedagogies can help support, explore challenges of integrating the arts and humanities into medical education and opportunities for how best to do that, and identify areas for further research. The report also provides examples of curricula that integrate arts and humanities in creative and effective ways to achieve a variety of outcomes. The methods and strategies of the AAMC FRAHME initiative appear in Appendix A.

*The **arts** teach creative means of expression, understanding of different perspectives, an awareness of knowledge and emotions throughout the human experience, and the shaping and sharing of perceptions through artistic creation and practices in the expressive world. — NASEM 2018*

Though categorizations differ, the humanities tend to include disciplines such as literature, history, philosophy, and art criticism and theory, while the arts embody creative expression through the visual and performing arts, crafts, and literary and media arts. The humanities often explore and engage lived experience in the human world. (Although ethics is considered a humanities discipline,[3] we do not address it here because we included it in *Behavioral and Social Science Foundations for Future Physicians.*[2])

*The **humanities** teach close reading practices as an essential tool, an appreciation for context across time and space, qualitative analysis of social structures and relationships, the importance of perspective, the capacity for empathic understanding, analysis of the structure of an argument … . — NASEM 2018*

According to a recent National Academies of Sciences, Engineering, and Medicine (NASEM) report, "The **humanities** teach close reading practices as an essential tool, an appreciation for context across time and space, qualitative analysis of social structures and relationships, the importance of perspective, the capacity for empathic understanding, analysis of the structure of an argument … ."[4] The domain of the fine and performing arts may include music, drama, dance, creative writing, visual arts, design, new media, and film. The NASEM report also noted: "The **arts** teach creative means of expression, understanding of different perspectives, an awareness of knowledge and emotions throughout the human experience, and the shaping and sharing of perceptions through artistic creation and practices in the expressive world."[4]

A working definition of the arts and humanities in medical education: Content or pedagogy derived from arts and humanities and integrated into the teaching and learning of medical students, trainees, and practicing physicians. The approaches and experiences with this education are often interprofessional, interdisciplinary, and co-designed to teach and sustain diverse competencies for better health outcomes for patients, communities, and populations.

AAMC

2. Introduction and Historical Context

American medical education and our broader, complex health care systems are evolving rapidly. New demands of the 21st century require that physicians adapt to rapid changes and advances in care delivery. The curricula designed to teach and assess medical students, residents, fellows, and fully licensed physicians require continuous improvement and adaptation to meet these new demands. **The arts and the humanities play a unique and not fully realized role in this educational process, and we strongly encourage increased integration of the arts and humanities into curricula across the continuum of medical education.** This report provides an overview of the current landscape of approaches that integrate arts and humanities into curricula and guidance about how to effect the integration. It is written for physician learners and for professionals teaching medical students (undergraduate medical education), resident and fellowship physicians (graduate medical education), and physicians in practice (continuing professional development).

What do we mean by the integration of arts and humanities in medicine?

Integrative educational models intentionally seek to "bridge the knowledge, modes of inquiry, and pedagogies from multiple disciplines ... within the context of a single course or program of study."[4] A landmark report published by NASEM in 2018[4] recommended that in our era of increasingly narrow specialization, higher education must intentionally develop models that integrate the arts and humanities with the sciences to meet the challenges and opportunities of the 21st century and to better prepare our learners for "work, life, and citizenship." This report, *The Integration of the Humanities and Arts with Sciences, Engineering, and Medicine in Higher Education: Branches from the Same Tree*, highlights the essential interconnectedness of all domains of inquiry and draws its title from Einstein's assertion that "all religion, arts, and sciences are branches from the same tree."

Integrated curricula in medical education have a long history, and their number has increased over the past decades.[5-7] However, most attention has focused on the integration of foundational and applied sciences at the medical school level in efforts to modify the traditional 2 + 2 structure (two years of basic, or foundational, sciences, then two years of clinical, or applied, sciences).[8] More recent efforts have been made to weave together these sciences with newer topics such as quality improvement, interprofessional teamwork, cultural humility, population health, and health policy.[8-11] We contend that the arts and humanities are intrinsically connected to teaching and learning in medicine, and pedagogical approaches should be woven into the fabric of 21st-century medical students' education, resident physicians' training, and physicians' ongoing development.

Arts and humanities integration within medical education curricula may employ a variety of art forms, including literature, poetry, theater, performing arts, and visual arts, as well as various pedagogical strategies that use these forms. The numerous goals for integrating arts and humanities within medical education include increasing certain nuanced capacities asserted by many scholars, such as tolerance of ambiguity and paradox, sensitivity to form in language, and comprehension of patient stories.[12-14] Other goals, cited in the NASEM report, include:

- Ingraining aspects of professionalism, empathy, and altruism.
- Enhancing clinical communication and observation skills.
- Increasing interprofessionalism and collaboration.
- Decreasing burnout and compassion fatigue.

How did we get here?

Dating back to ancient civilizations, the arts and humanities have been integral to the practice of medicine.[15] In Greek mythology, Apollo was the god of healing and diseases, music and poetry, truth and prophecy, and more, and it was to Apollo that Hippocrates dedicated his famous oath reminding us that "there is art to medicine as well as science."[16] The 20th century was marked by a rising predominance of science and technology in medicine and medical education. Abraham Flexner's influential, and controversial, 1910 report called for an educationally rigorous scientific base for medicine.[17] Practically, this brought about the traditional 2 + 2 curricular structure, as well as evidence-informed teaching and more rigorous assessment. Still, many notable physicians have upheld the essential need for interweaving humanistic practice and scientific rigor into the practice of medicine. William Osler, for example, called medicine "an old art [that] ... must be absorbed in the new science."[18]

After World War II, the ascendancy of science was supported in the United States by the emergence of the National Institutes of Health, replete with grant funding to support research in the basic sciences. In 1959, C.P. Snow, PhD, a famed scientist and novelist, delivered his "two cultures" lecture, which postulated that the intellectual life of all of Western society was split into two cultures — the sciences and the humanities — and this constituted a major barrier to solving the world's problems.[19] More recently, some have called for integrative models of learning in general and for the integration of arts and humanities with science in particular.[4]

The 1960s marked the emergence of the field of medical humanities, with many medical schools beginning to offer required or elective humanities courses. In 1967, the first department of humanities in any medical school was established at Penn State University College of Medicine. In 1969, the Society for Health and Human Values was founded, which championed humanities teaching in medical education and practice. With funding from the National Endowment for the Humanities, the society held convenings and provided guidance on integrating humanities into medical school curricula. In 1979, the *Journal of Medical Humanities* was established in the United States. Five years later, Eric Cassell, MD, prepared a report for the Hastings Center, *The Place of Humanities in Medicine*, which considered existing and emerging humanities programs within medical schools.[20]

The field of narrative medicine, pioneered by Rita Charon, MD, PhD, at Columbia University College of Physicians and Surgeons (now Vagelos College of Physicians and Surgeons), was developed beginning in the late 1990s as a way to cultivate empathy, reflection, professionalism, and trust in medicine.[21-23] This method uses close reading and writing to examine four of medicine's critical narrative situations: physician and patient, physician and self, physician and colleagues, and physician and society (see Section 5, page 22, for more details).

In 2000, *Medical Humanities* was established as a companion journal to the *Journal of Medical Ethics* and offered an additional publishing outlet for a disparate community of enthusiasts working largely in silos.[24] Beginning in 2010, the Project to Rebalance and Integrate Medical Education (PRIME) held a series of workshops to undertake a critical appraisal of the goals and objectives of medical humanities and bioethics teaching, and participants concurred that medical humanities integration was essential for professional development in medicine.[25,26]

In 2015, a group of physician educators and trainees founded Doctors Who Create to encourage and reward creativity in medicine (doctorswhocreate.com). This undergraduate, graduate, and continuing medical education (UME-GME-CME) team organized and hosted a Creativity in Medicine conference in 2019 at the Mütter Museum in Philadelphia, bringing together people from around the United States to share their original works through workshops, art and musical performances, storytelling, and more. Also in 2015, the Health Humanities Consortium was founded to promote "health humanities scholarship, education, and practices through interdisciplinary methods and theories that focus on the intersection of the arts and humanities, health, illness and healthcare."[27] The annual International Health Humanities Conference contributes to the sharing of best practices and the building of common theoretical underpinnings for this work.

An interdisciplinary national convening in 2016, the Art of Examination: Art Museums and Medical School Partnerships, brought together professionals at the Museum of Modern Art in New York to consider the current and future states of medical education and museum partnerships.[28] The forum included educators from 60 art museums and 60 medical schools who had existing partnerships dedicated to engaging medical learners with works of art. In recent years, the AAMC Group on Educational Affairs launched special interest groups in health humanities to foster communities of practice and explore the many ways the arts and humanities can inform health care.

Over the past decade, the vast majority of U.S. medical schools have incorporated arts and humanities to varying degrees, and many have found novel and foundational ways to ensure the arts and humanities are valued and incorporated. In the 2017-2018 academic year, 94% of medical schools reported having required or elective courses in medical humanities.[29] The content, pedagogy, evaluation, and degree of integration are highly variable, however. Many medical schools have begun to offer arts and humanities special interest tracks and scholarly concentrations, which often include the option to engage deeply in an arts or humanities domain.

Although the integration of arts and humanities at the GME and CME levels isn't yet common, it is growing at the premedical level. Medical school admissions committees seek to admit well-rounded humanistic learners to the field of medicine. The Liaison Committee for Medical Education (LCME®), for example, recommends that students preparing to study medicine should "acquire a broad undergraduate education that includes the study of the humanities, natural sciences, and social sciences."[30] Colleges and universities have seen significant growth in new medical humanities baccalaureate programs, including major and minor concentrations. According to researchers at Case Western Reserve University School of Medicine, over the past 20 years, the number of health humanities programs has increased nearly sevenfold, from 15 to 102, and another five programs are in development.[31]

3. The Fundamental Role of the Arts and Humanities in Medical Education and Physician Development

The needs of today's health care system call for skills and competencies that can be fostered, in part, through integrated arts and humanities curricular practices. These include communication, teaming, adaptability, creativity, critical thinking, empathy, social advocacy, and resiliency. Human suffering and illness arise within complex contexts, and a physician's ability to practice may be well served by exploration, construction of new ways of thinking, or even discovery of new questions or problems.[32,33] Effective engagement with the arts and humanities also supports professional identity formation in the practice of medicine.[34-37] Learner participation in integrative arts and humanities curricula may allow for deconstruction of silos of specialization.

Professional growth and transformation occur when we adopt the perspective of others through acts of sustained attention so we can represent and reflect on what we see, hear, or read, as well as when we develop the ability to think critically and compassionately about human dilemmas.[21,26,38,39] The cultivation of practical wisdom, or phronesis, leads to the ability to integrate one's deep fund of knowledge, ethical sensibilities, and emotional intelligence to know how to do the right thing in *this* circumstance, with *this* patient.[40,41]

Being a doctor requires continuous learning, unlearning, and relearning and being able to formulate good questions, put disparate concepts together, and innovate. Arts and humanities learning in medical education may affect *the ability to learn* in a truly integrative fashion. It allows learners to exercise the intellect and emotions in new ways and to see patterns in and make connections between seemingly distinct subjects.[42,43] The arts and humanities provide physicians, trainees, and other health care professionals with outlets for creative expression, meaning-making, and joy.[44-47] Engagement with the arts and humanities can support these essential abilities throughout the training and careers of physicians.

How are the arts and humanities integrated within medical education?

Arts and humanities have been integrated into medical education in many ways, from offering a single elective experience to fully integrating them across the entire program (Table 1). This continuum includes within-session, within-course, and within-program integration. The level of integration depends on the local curricula and desired learning outcomes.

Table 1. Approaches for Integrating Arts and Humanities Into Medical Education

Approach	Description	Example
Within-Session Integration	Arts and humanities experiences are included in an existing single session or learning activity.	**55-Word Stories** at a Society of Teachers of Family Medicine (STFM) Seminar[48]
Within-Course or Within-Rotation Integration	Arts and humanities experiences are included throughout an existing course or rotation.	**My Life, My Story Veterans Program** at VA medical centers[49] (See Section 5, page 24.)
Within-Program Integration	Arts and humanities experiences are included as a course or courses (elective or required) in an existing program.	**Medical Improv Selective** at Northwestern Feinberg School of Medicine[50] (See Section 5, page 23.)
Longitudinal Within-Program Integration	Arts and humanities experiences are included as a *longitudinal* track, thread, or course (elective or required) in an existing program.	**Literature and Medicine** at Georgetown University School of Medicine[51] (See Section 5, page 25.)

What role do these approaches play in competency-based education?

Competency-based education (CBE) is an emerging approach to health professions education that emphasizes learning *outcomes*, including competencies, rather than the process of teaching. Over the past 20 years, medical education has improved in many ways, including in how outcomes such as competencies are defined and used to guide teaching and learning. The alignment of approaches that integrate the arts and humanities with current health care needs and desired learner and physician outcomes is imperative. Integrative curricula result ideally in outcomes or competencies that are relevant and valued in academic medicine, such as the six general competencies listed below.

In 1999, the Accreditation Council for Graduate Medical Education (ACGME) and the American Board of Medical Specialties (ABMS) defined and adopted the six general competencies for practicing physicians, which remain prominent in today's medical education systems:[52]

- Medical knowledge.
- Patient care and procedural skills.
- Professionalism.
- Interpersonal and communication skills.
- Systems-based practice.
- Practice-based learning and improvement.

What are barriers to integration?

Increasing integrative arts and humanities curricula within academic medicine faces several barriers, including beliefs that the curriculum is "full" — there is no space for adding more — and that doing so would bring little or no meaningful value[39] and challenge the legacy of a dominant science emphasis. Thinking of curricular space through a lens of aggregation and not integration leads some people to argue there is no more room to add content or learning experiences. However, integrative approaches often remove redundancies and provide more efficient methods for teaching and learning than segregated approaches.[53]

What we value is shown, at least in part, by what we choose to support with funding, grants, calls for research and evaluation, and promotion criteria for teaching and scholarship. These expressions of value are key themes throughout this report, as is the need to better align values with more holistic approaches to teaching and learning.

What are key functions of integrative curricula?

The FRAHME initiative's commissioned scoping review led to an emerging theory of practice, the Prism Model.[54] Building on earlier conceptual work by Dennhardt et al.[55] and qualitative analysis of the published literature, the Prism Model addresses the following four functions of the arts and humanities in medical education: mastering skills, perspective-taking, personal insight, and social advocacy or sociocultural critique and change. In the Prism Model, each function is conceptualized as a lens in a prism that can help educators approach any domain they wish to teach (e.g., communication, empathy) in multiple ways, depending on which function is emphasized. Each function offers a different yet interrelated way of seeing arts and humanities teaching. The four functions are most powerful when used in combination, as a way to more fully recognize all pedagogical possibilities for arts- and humanities-based teaching in medical education.

The four functions proposed by the research team differ from the six general competencies (i.e., medical knowledge, patient care and procedural skills, professionalism, interpersonal and communication skills, systems-based practice, and practice-based learning and improvement). While the functions help focus one's approach to teaching and curriculum development in the arts and humanities, the competencies are broad, desired physician learning outcomes. Each competency can be taught in multiple ways, and the four functions provide a conceptual background for designing and executing ways to teach the competencies:

Mastering skills focuses on helping learners acquire the knowledge and skills relevant to clinical care. Examples of such skills include case presentation and reporting, communication, critical thinking, and ethical reasoning.

Perspective-taking focuses on making visible, through interaction and dialogue, the sometimes contradictory perspectives of people involved in clinical encounters, especially patients, and on enriching learners' own perspectives and attitudes in the process.

Personal insight focuses on fostering awareness of and reflection about inward processes and struggles, which contribute to professional identity formation, emotional growth, personal wellness, and resilience.

Social advocacy focuses on social issues and incites the learner to question, critique, and transform norms as well as potential inequities and injustices in health care and society more broadly. Examples include using arts and humanities to reveal and respond to issues such as a lack of access to health care, the social determinants of health, and equity, diversity, and inclusion.

Arts and humanities interventions can address many 21st-century health care challenges. The section below provides several examples of using arts and humanities interventions to foster teamwork and collaboration, support learner well-being and promote resilience, and adapt to and drive change. Addressing these challenges may serve several functions identified by Moniz et al.[54] For a step-by-step exercise in how to apply the model to curriculum design, see the Prism Exercise in the Moniz et al. paper. In summary, medical educators should ask:

1. What problem(s) are we trying to solve?
2. What are current competency gaps, and how is the program or curriculum addressing this problem now?
3. Which of the four functions suit these competencies? Are we working to improve skill, gain perspective, foster personal insight, or increase awareness of inequities? Can more than one function be addressed when different angles of a complex phenomenon are being considered?
4. What goals and objectives will address these gaps and functions?
5. What approaches or experiences — inclusive of pedagogy based in arts and humanities — can allow these goals and objectives to be achieved? Return to Step 2 and ask: Can the arts-and-humanities-based approaches enhance the existing program or curricula?
6. What evidence exists to support these approaches? What evidence can be gathered to evaluate the impact of the curriculum?
7. How does the new evidence gathered change the curriculum or the experience? What can be improved based on this information?

What are some examples of using arts and humanities interventions to foster teamwork and collaboration, resilience, and flexibility?

Foster Teamwork and Collaboration: In the past couple of decades, interprofessional collaborative practice has become central to safe and effective patient care. Atul Gawande, MD, notes that we continue to "train, hire, and pay doctors to be cowboys. But it's pit crews people need."[56] Physicians require ***perspective-taking*** of their teammates to learn to fully function in an interdependent manner. They need ***personal insight*** to reflect on their own attitudes and assumptions about hierarchy and the physician role, and they need to ***master skills*** of constructive communication and feedback. By engaging together in arts and humanities integrative curricula, entire clinical teams (e.g., attendings, students, nurses, and ward clerks) can more effectively translate learning into actual health care settings.[57]

An example of an integrative model that teaches teamwork to interprofessional learners and applies three lenses from the Prism Model is the Brigham and Women's Hospital Multidisciplinary Teambuilding Museum Workshops.[58] Beginning in 2009, these workshops have been a required component of an inpatient general medicine rotation. In addition to interns and residents, teams include attending physicians, nurses, medical students, pharmacy students, physical therapists, and care coordinators. The sessions are designed around engagement with works of art and are explicitly designed to "break down hierarchical relationships, to improve constructive discussion [***master skills***] and understand differing perspectives [***perspective-taking***], to stimulate awareness [***personal insight***] of how the group works together as a team, and to be fun."[58]

The University of Wisconsin-Madison offers another example of an integrative arts-based curriculum: using improvisational theater techniques to teach empathy to teams of health professions students.[59] Their course includes assigned reading, sharing experiences with improv in their daily lives, and playing improv games. Over the course of six weeks, students are taught to observe and listen well (***master skills***), take others' perspectives (***perspective-taking***), and focus their immediate reactions on furthering the goals of the group as a whole (***social advocacy***).

Support Learner Well-being and Promote Resilience: Physician burnout, depression, and suicide have many root causes, including uncertainty, long hours, and bearing witness to human suffering.[60] In addition, the current system of financing and delivery of health care creates contradictory and values-challenging incentives for physicians and health care systems. Watching their role models navigate the painful choices that follow — such as the challenge of controlling costs while providing quality patient-centered care or engaging with the patient while documenting an exam in the electronic patient record — may have a negative impact on learners. Physicians have begun to describe these dilemmas as "morally injurious" double binds in which clinical engagement requires witnessing, perpetrating, or failing to prevent the transgression of deeply held moral beliefs about the role of healing and health care.[61] Well-designed arts and humanities curricula can support renewal and restoration of meaning, as well as help learners navigate inherent paradoxes and tensions in the learning and practice of medicine today.[62]

Personal insight into one's own maladaptive behaviors and coping strategies can be supported by arts and humanities interventions.[63] The Stanford Medicine WellMD Center promotes the practice of prioritizing community in an institution as part of a "culture of wellness," one of three components of professional fulfillment. To build community for Stanford physicians and trainees, the center engages in several arts and humanities initiatives, including a literature and medicine dinner series in which participants reflect on the challenges and rewards of being a doctor; an annual symposium titled Medicine and the Muse featuring artists, writers, and performers; the Stanford Medicine Music Network, which connects healers, musicians, and music lovers; and Wednesday Night Writes, a weekly writing group that helps attendees hone their voice, tone, and structure skills.[64]

An example of an integrative approach that fosters resilience and enhances sense of purpose (***personal insight***) is a collaborative program between the University of Colorado Anschutz Medical Campus and local arts organizations.[65] Supported by the National Endowment for the Arts as an NEA Arts Research Lab, the intervention is for critical care and emergency medicine professionals who have at least one symptom of burnout. The program integrates visual arts therapy, music therapy, dance/movement therapy, and creative writing/poetry, and it uses qualitative, mixed-method, and randomized controlled study designs to evaluate effectiveness.

Another example of an integrative approach is Transforming Moral Injury Across the Professions: Cultivating Moral Resilience Through Reflective Writing and Contemplative Practice, developed by the Braxton Institute for Sustainability, Resiliency and Joy in partnership with the Volunteers of America (VOA) and the Los Angeles County Department of Mental Health.[66] For "clinicians, war-fighters, chaplains, social workers, emergency workers, community organizers, VOA ministers and anyone interested in cultivating practical tools for sustainable self-care," the program is intended to help the healer heal the self not by diminishing or minimizing moral adversity, but by naming it and addressing it (***personal insight***). Participants learn multiple forms of exploration and meaning-making that realistically support building moral resilience and recovery from moral adversity.

Improve Flexibility and Ability to Drive Change: Change is inevitable in health care. Even a quarter century ago, we could not have predicted the impact of technology on health care, the need to adapt to new care-delivery models during a public health pandemic such as COVID-19, or the transition to the focus on systems-based practice. The physician of today and tomorrow must be able to drive as well as adapt to change. Critical engagement with the arts and humanities may help make visible the deep social forces that lead to human suffering and disparities in health.[67-69] The arts and humanities may provide examples, tools, and inspiration for individuals and groups to master new leadership skills, thoughtfully challenge the status quo, and engage in ***social advocacy***.

An integrative model that addresses adapting to and driving change was piloted as the opening session at an Agency for Healthcare Research and Quality (AHRQ) conference to establish a research agenda on the emotional impact of medical harm.[70] They used visual images and metaphors as gateways to personal reflections among diverse stakeholders. Themes identified included chaos and turmoil, profound isolation, organizational denial, moral injury and betrayal, negative effects on families and communities, importance of relational skills, and healing effects of human connection (***personal insight, social advocacy***). The exercise invited storytelling, enabled psychological safety, and fostered the development of an action agenda.[71]

Johns Hopkins School of Medicine uses humanities lessons on the history of medicine to examine comparisons between anti-Asian sentiments during the current COVID-19 pandemic and the xenophobia of Cape Town during the bubonic plague. Students gain an understanding of appropriate and inappropriate health policy responses (***social advocacy***) when they learn that in 1901, the plague provided an opportunity to remove Black citizens from the European population, which served as the foundation for apartheid.[72]

What are deliberate pedagogies for integrative curricula?

Having good clinical skills or expert content knowledge does not necessarily make a physician a good teacher. Most learners do not emerge from medical training as well-equipped educators, facilitators, or preceptors. Faculty development is important to all who take on the role of educator, including those who integrate arts and humanities curricula. Educators' own assumptions about, and personal experiences with, teaching and learning will most certainly influence the effectiveness of using educational strategies that employ the arts and humanities.[73]

The faculty development necessary to achieve integration requires time, funding, and other forms of institutional support, such as recognition toward tenure and promotion. The NASEM consensus report recommends that institutions working to implement integrative curricular models set aside resources for the hiring, research, teaching activities, and professional development of faculty who can teach integrative courses or programs (Recommendation 3).[4]

The NASEM report also calls for deliberate pedagogy and attention to the nuances of successful interdisciplinary collaboration. Integrative arts and humanities curricula add an additional layer of complexity to pedagogy, and for certain educational goals and contexts, educators should engage with specific and established expertise within the arts and humanities. Medical educators should consider nontraditional partners and collaborate with colleagues from university departments outside medicine (e.g., departments of education, psychology, history, literary studies, philosophy, anthropology, fine arts). Guiding learners through critical analysis of literary texts, for example, may best be accomplished with faculty trained in literature. Certain models involving coproduction and cofacilitation have been successful, where the physician-partner is responsible for helping learners "translate" the art experience into relevant learning for clinical practice.[74,75]

In addition to teaching, facilitating, and precepting, educators need skills to design effective integrated curricula and evaluate them. Educational activities should be informed by theories of adult learning and sound curricular design,[8,76] including how to make learning relevant and experiential, assess and draw on prior knowledge, engage learners' curiosity, differentiate for learner needs, design curricula, and assess learning outcomes. From the great diversity of approaches to integrating arts and humanities described in the literature, common elements emerge: Exposure to the unique qualities of the arts (e.g., metaphorical, complex, ambiguous, universal) is necessary, but not sufficient, to making learning relevant to medical education goals, and educator expertise must explicitly inform methods of engagement, meaning-making strategies, and translation of learning into actual clinical skills.[77]

What are effective methods for study and evaluation?

A detailed description of research and evaluation methods for arts and humanities integration is beyond the scope of this report. However, we would be remiss not to explore the fundamental need for a sound scholarly approach to the design, delivery, and evaluation of integrative approaches. *Educational research* is a social science defined as the "scientific field of study that examines education and learning processes and the human attributes, interactions, organizations, and institutions that shape educational outcomes. Education research embraces the full spectrum of rigorous methods appropriate to the questions being asked and also drives the development of new tools and methods."[78] Consequently, research about integrative arts and humanities curricula should embrace the "full spectrum" of scholarly approaches, including qualitative and mixed methods (Table 2).

Program evaluation is "the systematic collection of information about the activities, characteristics, and outcomes of programs to make judgments about the program, improve program effectiveness, and/or inform decisions about future program development."[79] Many academic educators conduct both research and evaluation, which may overlap in rigor and methods. Both are concerned with gathering evidence to support the intended outcomes. However, research focuses on creating new generalizable knowledge, proving hypotheses or theories, and determining which factors lead to certain effects or outcomes, while program evaluation focuses on determining how to improve a specific local program or curriculum.

Evidence-based practices to support the effectiveness of our educational interventions and methods are a cornerstone of medical education. How do we know an intervention is effective? What is the impact of an integrative curriculum on learning outcomes? The answers depend on how we define *evidence*. Academic medicine has traditionally defined it in quantitative terms, such as by achievement test scores. Although other forms of evidence, such as perspective-taking or empathic practice, are more difficult to measure, they remain important outcomes for teaching and learning in medicine. The evidence gathered should align with the intended learning outcomes and, therefore, qualitative or mixed methods may be most appropriate for evaluating many integrative arts and humanities curricula.

The AAMC FRAHME-commissioned scoping review described here and elsewhere found persistent gaps in educational program evaluation and learner assessment.[80] Additionally, the NASEM report found wide variability in the quality of published research on the outcomes associated with arts and humanities integration.[4] We support NASEM's strong encouragement of the development and use of rigorous research and evaluation methods when integrating the arts and humanities in science-based fields: "developers of integrative programs and courses should include a strong evaluation component to measure the effectiveness of integrative models on students' learning and workforce readiness" (Recommendation 1B).[4]

Whether evaluating the impact of an arts and humanities intervention on an individual learner or the overall effectiveness of a curricular innovation, we must begin by clearly identifying the outcomes the intervention is designed to achieve and assigning the appropriate assessment method or methods. For example, if we seek to learn whether an integrative arts curriculum leads to more precise interpretation of radiographic imaging by students, a quantitative measure may be most suitable. If, however, we seek to understand how learners develop empathy, then observations, interviews, narrative analyses, case studies, and other qualitative methods are likely to be most suitable.

Mixing relevant methods will allow for greater flexibility and more robust evaluation outcomes.[81] For example, a published instrument may be used to measure a characteristic of interest (e.g., empathy or tolerance of ambiguity) along with participants' observations and interviews. Qualitative methods are often used initially to gain a deeper understanding of learner experience or to develop theory, which may later lead to new experimental designs. Longitudinal studies with comparison or control groups will likely be needed and institutionally supported to establish arts and humanities integration as standard in medical education. Many medical educators envision these different research and evaluation methods as complementary and perhaps sequential, leading to a generalizable body of research.

A related and important consideration in understanding the effectiveness of our interventions is how we define *research* and *scholarship*. Beginning in the late 1990s, higher education began to expand its definition of scholarship to recognize the rigor of discovery, integration, application, and teaching (Table 2). Before this movement, which was initiated by Ernest Boyer and the Carnegie Foundation for the Advancement of Teaching,[82] the academic medicine community expected teaching to be part of academic citizenship and integral, but insufficient, for academic promotion. The community of academic medicine in particular, and higher education in general, now views the educators' roles, expectations, and criteria differently. As Boyer stated, the faculty are a "mosaic of talent," and their scholarly efforts should be recognized and developed fully.[82]

Table 2. General Types of Scholarship in U.S. Higher Education

Approach	Description
Discovery	Building new knowledge through traditional research methods.
Integration	Making connections across disciplines, placing specialties in a broader context, and integrating those connections for new knowledge.
Application	Applying existing research findings, expertise, and innovations to remedy societal problems tied directly to one's field of knowledge.
Teaching	Researching and evaluating teaching models, methods, and programs to optimize learning outcomes.

Source: Boyer EL. Scholarship Reconsidered: Priorities of the Professoriate. *Princeton, NJ: Carnegie Foundation for the Advancement of Teaching;1990.*

In 2006, the AAMC Group on Educational Affairs (GEA) convened a consensus conference to explore and advance the construct of teaching as scholarship.[76] Among the questions addressed were: What are the criteria for educational scholarship? What are the necessary resources and infrastructure required to support educators as scholars? The GEA agreed that a scholarly approach to education required systematic design, implementation, evaluation, and redesign informed by the literature and best practices in the field. A work of teaching scholarship or a scholarly product must be accessible to the education community, presented in a form that others can build on, and be available to peers to review using accepted criteria.

Careful attention to how we measure and report the impact or the effectiveness of educational interventions will prevent overly broad generalizations or claims. Statements that claim exposure to the arts and humanities "improves well-being" or "increases empathy" lead to many questions: Which art form or humanities modality? What sort of engagement, in what context, for how long? Effective education research and evaluation methods can help address these and other questions as we improve our understanding of these integrative practices.

Careful attention to how we measure and report the impact or effectiveness of these interventions will also help us understand how differences within their design and delivery affect outcomes. Given that the arts and humanities include many modalities (e.g., literature, visual arts, music), we should be cautious in examining their effects or when making causal claims. In other words, we should avoid lumping together art forms and instructional approaches or pedagogies in our research and evaluation processes. Similarly, efforts to identify the unique impacts these interventions may have are important. When comparing effects of educational arts and humanities interventions on outcomes, we should pay attention to differentiating the plausible alternative explanations for those outcomes.

4. Current Landscape and Research Needs

What is the scope of published literature on arts and humanities in medical education?

In 2019, the AAMC commissioned a team from the University of Western Ontario, Penn State College of Medicine, and Mount Saint Vincent University to complete a scoping review on **how and why the arts and humanities are being used to educate physicians and interprofessional learners across the developmental spectrum,** from UME to GME to CME (see Appendix B).

This section summarizes that review. For a more detailed description of findings, see the team's related publications.[54,80] The search strategy yielded 769 works — journal articles, books, book chapters, dissertations, and theses — published between January 1991 and June 2019. The inclusion criteria were:

- Experiences from premedical education through continuing medical education.
- Programs for physicians or physician learners, including those with other interprofessional learners.
- Elective and required experiences.
- Qualitative and quantitative research, as well as descriptive and conceptual papers.
- English language material.

Record and Method Types: Most records were journal articles (n = 610, 79%), followed by book chapters (n = 144, 19%), books (n = 10, 1%), and dissertations or theses (n = 5, 1%). Most records were conceptual (n = 294, 38%) or descriptive (n = 255, 33%) pieces, followed by empirical studies (n = 169, 22%) and reviews (n = 51, 7%).

Descriptive records included pieces that described 1) courses or initiatives at medical schools and 2) how a specific humanities subject or art form can be used within medical education. Of the empirical works, qualitative studies (n = 77, 45%) dominated, followed closely by studies that reported both qualitative and quantitative results (n = 60, 36%); there were comparatively fewer quantitative studies (n = 32, 19%). Of the reviews, one-third were described by authors as literature reviews (n = 17, 33%). Others were described as systematic reviews (n = 4, 8%), scoping reviews (n = 3, 6%), and narrative reviews (n = 3, 6%). Almost half the reviews were categorized as "other" (n = 24, 47%), which included systematic listings in response to a research question and works described as a "review" without further specifying type. Only 73 (10%) of the 769 records described educational programming or interventions that involved physicians with other health professionals.

Art Forms and Humanities Subjects: The largest number of records fell into the category "**arts and humanities general**" (n = 170, 22%), which referred to records that discussed the "arts and humanities" as a general field and records that listed various art forms or humanities subjects without focused attention on any one (e.g., a combination of narrative medicine, creative writing workshops, and learners submitting assignments in narrative, poetry, song, or video form). A significant subset of records involved the **literary arts**, focusing on the use of literature in medical education (n = 197, 26%), followed by **reflective writing** (n = 119, 15%), **narrative medicine** (n = 86, 11%), and "other" types of writing such as **creative writing and poetry** (n = 61, 8%). **Visual art** was the focus of 82 records (11%), almost half of which were about learners observing the art and a quarter of which were about learners creating the art. **Theater and drama** was discussed in 70 (9%) records. These records were divided almost evenly into engaging learners by observing or reading, by performing, or by doing both activities. Sixty-seven records (9%) focused on educating medical learners using **film and television**. Of these, the vast majority (n = 63, 94%) focused on learners engaging with film or television by watching it (rather than creating it). Twenty-one (3%) records focused on using **music** to educate physicians. Of these, half engaged learners in listening to music, such as listening to jazz to help them develop improvisational communication skills for medical encounters with patients; another five records (25%) engaged learners in creating music. Seventeen records (2%) focused on **comics and graphic novels**; 10 of those (59%) engaged learners through reading, one (6%) involved learners creating comics or graphic novels, and five (29%) had learners both reading and creating comics and graphic novels. Eleven records (1%) described using **Visual Thinking Strategies (VTS)** with medical learners, an approach that facilitates identifying and examining various perspectives and emotions elicited by the art. A very small number of records described using **history** ($n = 6$, <1%) and **religion** ($n = 5$, <1%).

Learner Type: The team conducted descriptive statistics on a subset of the data ($n = 424$) pertaining to descriptive ($n = 255$, 60%) and empirical ($n = 169$, 40%) records only. They found the arts and humanities programming in **undergraduate medical education** dominated the data set ($n = 245$, 58%), the focus of more than half the records. **Postgraduate medical education** occupied less than a quarter of records ($n = 73$, 17%). **Premedical education** ($n = 20$, 5%) and **continuing medical education** ($n = 13$, 3%) received minimal attention in the literature reviewed.

Evaluation and Assessment: In terms of **program evaluation**, arts and humanities educational programming was evaluated in 226 records (53%). In about one-quarter of records, there wasn't enough information to determine whether evaluation occurred. Learners were assessed for their participation in arts and humanities educational programming about one-quarter of the time ($n = 116$, 27%). Most often, learners were either not assessed or the authors did not report assessing them ($n = 298$, 70%).

Pedagogical Functions: A qualitative analysis of the pedagogical functions for 769 records describing the integrative arts-and-humanities-based experiences grouped them according to these functions:

- Arts and humanities for mastering skills.
- Arts and humanities for perspective-taking.
- Arts and humanities for personal insight.
- Arts and humanities for social advocacy.

Although these approaches overlap (many reported multiple functions), nearly half the records fell within the "mastering skills" ($n = 163$, 21%) and "perspective-taking" functions ($n = 158$, 21%).

What are research gaps and areas for future study?

The scoping review, by design, did not critique the quality of the published literature, and, as with teaching and learning more broadly, the peer-reviewed literature may not accurately reflect practice. Nevertheless, the review process identified gaps also found in other reports and findings. First, relatively few records described learning experiences designed for premedical, GME, and CME learners or interprofessional education and contexts. Only 10% of records included both medical learners and learners from other professions. Voices from patients, learners, artists, museum educators, and humanities scholars were lacking from the educational programs and initiatives. Only 30% of the records were explicitly framed by theory, and a small majority reported evaluating the approach or assessing the learners. Filling these gaps would help advance our understanding and future practice.

What factors support the growth of arts and humanities integration?

Medical school and health care system support is essential to the success of arts and humanities integration. Today, much of the curriculum development and teaching in this domain is driven by individual faculty interest, with many passionate educators volunteering their personal time. Institutions should adopt the following actions to support the integration of arts and humanities into medical education:

1. Value the unique contribution of integrative arts and humanities approaches to medical education and physician development.
2. Promote and support broad types of faculty scholarship, including those that advance integrative arts and humanities practices.
3. Adopt a broad definition of scholarship for appointment, promotion, and tenure for medical school faculty.
4. Collaborate and coproduce curricula with professionals within and outside medicine.
5. Practice integrative (not isolated or siloed) models of curriculum design and delivery.
6. Offer faculty development in teaching, curriculum design, and assessment methods.
7. Establish funding sources within medical schools and through external channels such as foundations.

Recommendations for Advancing Scholarship

- Engage more diverse perspectives and voices in the literature by including those of learners, patients, and arts and humanities scholars.
- Ground integrative approaches in best evidence and theory.
- Increase interprofessional and multidisciplinary integrative approaches.
- Increase evaluation of and research on integrative curricular approaches.
- Increase research on the impact of arts and humanities integrative approaches on premedical, UME, GME, and CME learners and settings.

5. Examples of Integrative Approaches

There are many creative approaches to integrating the arts and humanities into medical education, and this section just begins to convey their possible goals, impacts, complexity, and creativity. It includes a summary of numerous approaches (Table 3) and brief descriptions of 13 examples of integrative curricula across the developmental continuum and the country. Each example's prominent content area or method is included in parentheses with its title. For more in-depth practical strategies for integrating the arts and humanities into medical education, see the FRAHME Digital Guidebook, available at aamc.org/FRAHME/Guidebook.

Table 3. Select Art Forms and Humanities Subjects: Content Areas and Methods for Teaching and Learning in Medicine

Art Form or Subject	Possible Extensions to Teaching and Learning in Medicine
Literature	A group of health professionals reads and discusses fiction and nonfiction literature that informs clinical practice, teaching, and learning.
Narrative medicine	Students participate in facilitated, small-group sessions of "close reading," learning how to thoughtfully and critically analyze a text and translate learnings to close listening with patients.
Theater and drama	Students practice active improvisation techniques that demonstrate listening without interruption and judgment.
Film and television	Students and patients view a film about patients' experiences with health and discuss inequities in care, bias, and stigma.
Music	Faculty take lessons by music teachers about effective coaching, observation, lifelong learning, feedback techniques, mindfulness, and more.
History	Interprofessional learners read and discuss seminal works about the historical context of race and the effects of institutional and structural racism on social determinants of health.
Religion and spirituality	Residents engage in "reflection rounds," a small-group activity in which learners consider the influence of patients' spiritual or religious beliefs on their illness experience.
Dance and movement	Students engage in dance and movement exercises to express emotion, reduce stress, and connect with patients.
Reflective writing	Students write reflective statements to learn from a critical incident or construct written tributes to anatomical donors and share them with the donors' family members.
Creative writing and poetry	Students and residents write, share, and discuss 55-word creative stories about impactful experiences.
Visual arts and thinking strategies	Interprofessional health care clinicians and learners view a work of visual art and engage in a facilitated discussion about the work, making connections to their own clinical practice.
Comics and graphic novels	Students create and share their own stories about formative experiences in creative comic form.

Training the Eye by Joel Katz, MD (Visual Arts)

Training the Eye: Improving the Art of Physical Diagnosis is a spring semester course for first-year medical students at Harvard Medical School. The course goals are to make careful looking a habit, to learn to link form and function, to recognize one's own biases, and to enjoy local art museums. This 10-session course takes place across three settings: the classroom, the art museum, and the clinic. Each session pairs a visual concept (e.g., form, balance, movement) to related aspects of the physical examination (e.g., breathing, cranial nerves, gait). Throughout the course, students practice skills of careful looking at both art and patients, thus enhancing observation, clinical reasoning, and communication skills related to physical diagnosis. Additional sessions cover the neurobiology of vision, a life drawing session, and Visual Thinking Strategies training, where, in facilitated discussions, students are invited to articulate what they observe, provide evidence for those observations, and make collaborative interpretations.

Narrative Medicine by Rita Charon, MD, PhD (Narrative Medicine)

Narrative medicine is a scholarly discipline based on literary and narrative theory, close reading, phenomenological inquiry, and creative principles that fortifies clinical practices of all health disciplines with ways to honor the stories of people who seek and give care. Created at Columbia University in 2000, the Narrative Medicine Program offers clinicians both conceptual frameworks and practical methods for developing egalitarian and intersubjective relationships with patients and colleagues toward both health care justice and effective health care.

Columbia University offers an MS degree in narrative medicine and an online Certification of Professional Achievement in Narrative Medicine and provides required curricula for 10 of Columbia's health professions schools. Intensive training weekends are held two or three times a year in New York City and elsewhere. Narrative Medicine West partners Columbia with the Kaiser Permanente Medical School and the Keck School of Medicine of the University of Southern California in Los Angeles. Partnerships between Columbia and universities and clinical institutions are growing in U.S. cities and in Milan, Paris, Istanbul, Mainz, Tokyo, Copenhagen, Odense, and elsewhere; these partnerships are giving rise to narrative medicine courses and electives that give students and clinicians the opportunity to write about and reflect on clinical experiences.

The Art of Communication by Karen Novak, DDS, PhD (Visual Arts)

The Summer Health Professions Education Program (SHPEP) at the McGovern Medical School at the University of Texas Health Science Center at Houston hosts 80 scholars per year for a six-week academic enhancement experience. Funded through the Robert Wood Johnson Foundation, this program serves undergraduate college students from diverse racial and ethnic groups, rural areas, and economically disadvantaged backgrounds who are interested in medicine, dentistry, or other health professions. One of the enrichment courses is the Art of Communication, which includes a session titled "The Art of Observation." In this session, students visit the Museum of Fine Arts, Houston, where they work on their observation and verbal communication skills. The students first view a portrait — for up to 20 minutes — then a museum docent describes the artist's concept of the art. Differences between their observations and the artist's concept are discussed. In a follow-up session, students view portraits or photos of actual patients and reflect on their observations: What do they perceive about the patient and their potential condition or disease? A physician describes the real condition and outcome of that patient. Through both processes, students learn the importance of closely observing their patients, that a cursory assessment is often misleading, and that a detailed look is often enlightening.

Playing Doctor by Katie Watson, JD (Theater and Drama)

Playing Doctor is a seminar created at Northwestern University Feinberg School of Medicine (NUFSM) in 2002. It begins with the observation that both physicians and theatrical improvisers must prepare for unpredictability and a barrage of new "scene partners" seeking to co-create shared stories and to agree on actions. Experts in both fields must learn to listen and observe, then respond and act, in stressful or confusing circumstances, and they both need superior team skills to flourish. Therefore, medical improv borrows principles and methods from improvisational theater and adapts them to medicine in active exercises designed to strengthen cognitive flexibility, emotional honesty, professionalism, and clear communication with patients and teammates.
The primary goal is to develop concrete skills and attitudes that embrace discovery, spontaneity, humility, confidence, and collaboration. Although medical improv has nothing to do with being funny, the method generates abundant laughter and camaraderie that has secondary benefits for wellness and humanism. NUFSM medical students are required to take a medical humanities "selective" (five weekly two-hour sessions) in both their first and second years, and Playing Doctor is one of 10 to 20 options they may choose from.

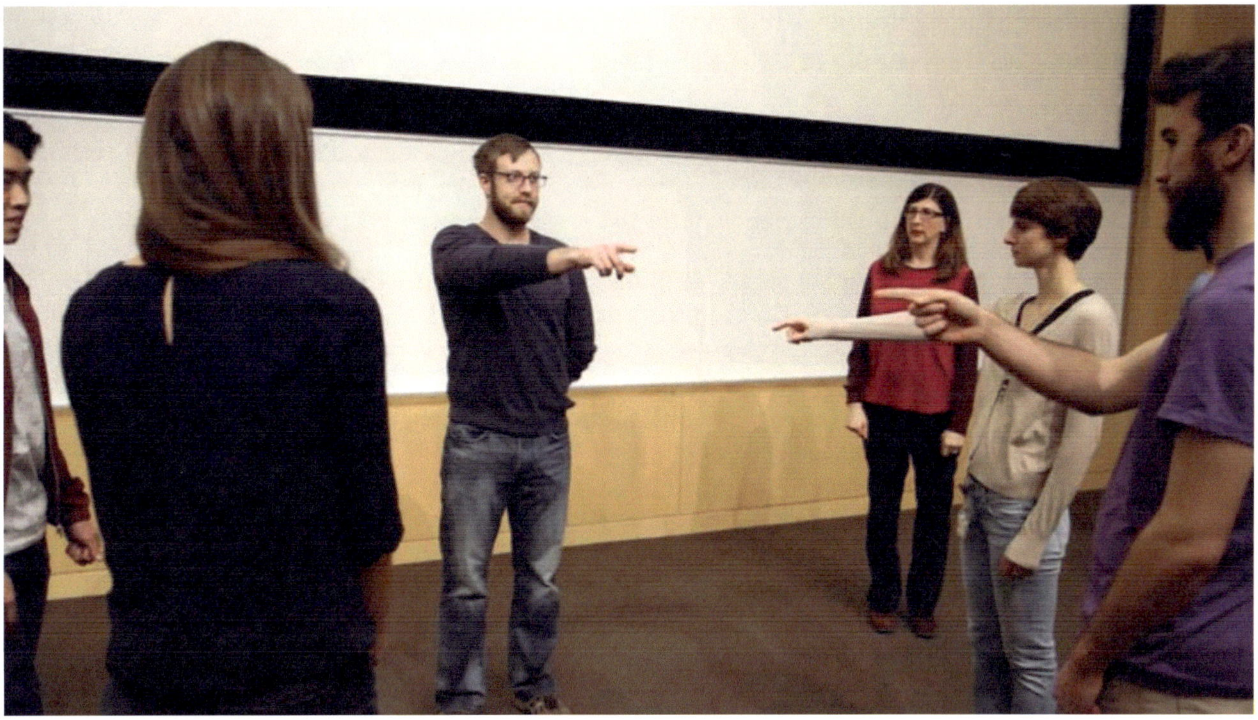

Katie Watson, JD, (in red) leads future physicians at Northwestern University in an exercise she says could make medical handoffs smoother. Courtesy of Jim Brucker.

My Life, My Story by Susan Nathan, MD (Reflective Writing)

In the My Life, My Story (MLMS)[49] program, created within Veterans Affairs medical centers, veterans are interviewed about their life stories by undergraduate and graduate trainees from diverse health professions. Learners work with veterans of all ages and states of health to craft their stories into concise, first-person narratives, review each story with the veteran, and, with the veteran's permission, enter it into a prominent place in the electronic medical record. The program serves two aims: bringing the veteran's story to the forefront of their care and enhancing learners' competencies in patient-centered care through a sharp focus on knowing the whole person.

MLMS has been integrated into the clinical education experience at VA Boston Healthcare System (VABHS) across various settings, including outpatient, inpatient hospice, and acute, postacute, and long-term care. The process is structured around an interview guide, detailed step-by-step instructions, a debrief guide for preceptors, and other materials. Although the overall process is structured, the experience can be tailored to meet the needs of the veteran, the learner, and the educational or clinical setting.

Medical Readers' Theater by Todd Savitt, PhD, and Sheena Eagan, MPH, PhD (Theater and Drama)

In 1988, Brody School of Medicine at East Carolina University developed a medical readers' theater program, still in use today, that educates health care students and professionals about social and ethical issues in medicine and, simultaneously, establishes a dialogue about these issues with the citizens of eastern North Carolina.

The concept is simple: adapt (with author permission) short stories about medicine to a script, invite health professions students to "perform" (i.e., read a character's lines while seated) the stories to public and medical audiences, and hold postperformance discussions with the audience and cast. The impact of these stories and discussions is often profound for both performers and audience members. Future health care providers hear the thoughts of future patients (and their peers and teachers), and audience members can voice ideas and feelings about ethical and social issues related to how medicine is practiced.

Jazz and the Art of Medicine by Paul Haidet, MD (Music)

One of the key features of high-quality medical communication is its improvisational nature. While communication training in medical school mostly focuses on basic skills in isolation (e.g., "history-taking" algorithms, how to break bad news), the messiness, uncertainty, and time pressure of real-world medical practice require practitioners be able to improvise and apply basic skills, patient by patient, in unique and creative ways.

In Jazz and the Art of Medicine, a course at Penn State College of Medicine, senior-level students learn that such real-time translation of basic communication elements is also what jazz musicians do when they play together. Like medicine, jazz uses basic communicative building blocks that need to be applied during the unscripted and emergent environment of the bandstand. During the course, students examine examples of improvisation from jazz and engage in discussion, reflection, and practice. Each learner creates a personal plan for continually practicing and building communication skills as they practice medicine in their chosen specialties, resulting in a progression from learning communication skills to becoming skilled communicators.

Literature and Medicine by Dan Marchalik, MD (Literature)

The Georgetown University School of Medicine Literature and Medicine Track is a four-year program rooted in literature and the medical humanities. The track aims to improve students' narrative competency and communication skills and to encourage the practice of self-reflection. In many ways, it functions to improve students' well-being and help combat burnout.

Starting in their first year of medical school, students join a monthly group discussion about various works of contemporary fiction, most of which do not have a primary medical focus. Students can meet with authors and explore other forms of medical humanities at local institutions such as the National Gallery of Art. During the clinical years, students participate in Medical Noon Conference — a journal club that focuses on works written by physicians. Most important, each student completes a capstone project rooted in the medical humanities before they graduate. Past projects include creating an obituary-writing program for anatomy lab and a monthly *BMJ* online book club and publishing both scholarly and mass-media articles in outlets such as *JAMA* and the *Washington Post*.

History of Medicine by Jeremy Greene, MD, PhD (History)

Like several other schools of medicine in North America, the Johns Hopkins School of Medicine expects all students to contribute to the development of medical knowledge through independent mentored research during the first two years of study. Unlike most other schools, however, Johns Hopkins has developed a scholarly concentration in the history of medicine that places this humanistic discipline on a par with the basic sciences and clinical research. Based in the Johns Hopkins Institute of the History of Medicine — the oldest and largest center for research in the history of medicine in the English-speaking world — this 16-month program trains medical students in the methods of literature-based, archive-based, and oral-historical research, as well as the approaches used in applying historical analysis to the present day. Students are paired with a faculty historian mentor for their independent research project in a field of their choosing. Those projects, involving fieldwork over five continents and narratives that stretch from the Middle Ages to the 21st century, have resulted in publications for clinical, historical, public health, and popular audiences and long-lasting involvement with history as a mode of humanistic engagement in clinical practice.

Documentary Film by Maren Monsen, MD (Film and Television)

Documentary film can be a powerful teaching tool because it gives viewers a chance to walk in someone else's shoes. At Stanford University School of Medicine, documentary film with facilitation is integrated throughout the curriculum and across the continuum, from UME through CME. To create a shared experience, faculty screen the films during class. Then, using a facilitator's guide that incorporates data and historical information, faculty work with small groups to discuss how this window into another person's life changes the students' perspective.

Premed students in a global health course watch *The Revolutionary Optimists*, a 50-minute film that follows a group of children in the slums of Kolkata over three years as they fought to bring clean water and vaccines to their community. In biochemistry and genetics courses for preclinical medical students, the short films *Hailey* and *Jack* are used as case studies of how the genetic disorders VLCADD and OTC deficiency affect patients and their families. In a cultural competence block, medical students and residents watch *Worlds Apart*, a series of short films that tell the stories of four culturally diverse patients and families faced with critical medical decisions as they navigate the health care system. Another film, *Hold Your Breath*, follows a devout Muslim immigrant who faces possible death from stomach cancer as cultural and linguistic confusions complicate his treatment in an American hospital.

Dance for All People by Rachel Balaban (Dance and Movement)

Artists and Scientists as Partners (ASaP) at Brown University is an innovative and interdisciplinary two-semester program where undergraduate (mostly premed) students study and work with both medical and arts practitioners to foster creative, integrative health practices. Faculty aim to help students understand the impact art has on people with neurological disorders, specifically Parkinson's disease and autism spectrum disorder.

Integrated into the curriculum is a two-month community-engagement experience called DAPpers (Dance for All People) inspired by the Mark Morris Dance Group. Adults with Parkinson's disease join students for weekly classes. Movement challenges provide a chance to engage in a holistic, nonmedicalized program to enhance wellness and quality of life, offering preprofessional doctors a window into the power of the arts to heal. DAPpers also introduces premed students to the value of self-care and empathy as they enter the medical profession, creating a pathway of training to increase physician empathy and decrease burnout. In addition to the classes, students partner with older dancers for interviews and weekly conversations. The relationships formed through this intergenerational community become meaningful for all participants and address some of the isolation and loneliness often felt by both populations.

The College Colloquium by Quentin Eichbaum, MD, PhD, MPH, MFA (Mixed)

The College Colloquium at Vanderbilt University School of Medicine is a required course with the broad goal of developing students into "flexible thinkers and agile learners with the mindful capacity for cognitive and emotional monitoring and regulation."[83] First-year medical students join weekly, two-hour sessions on meta-neurocognitive topics such as how we think, learn, decide, change, and reflect; how we tell stories; how we attend and pay attention; what it's like to be wrong and to make mistakes; and how we cope and gain resilience. Each session is preceded by a facilitated small-group discussion in which students examine various perspectives and learn how to disagree respectfully with one another, monitor and regulate their thinking and emotions, and (re)calibrate their views. Students also write critical reflection papers.

The colloquium is evaluated with a number of methods, including essay-style questions appearing within other course exams. In later years, students remark how their learning from the course helped them in problematic clinical encounters, with cognitive biases, stress, and medical error, and with developing resilience.

The Art of Medicine by Allison Bickett, PhD, and Mary Hall, MD (Visual Arts)

The Art of Medicine is an innovative collaboration between Atrium Health and the Bechtler Museum of Modern Art in Charlotte, N.C., originally designed and offered by Lisa Howley, lead author of this publication. It is the first program to combine the Balint method of "doctor-patient relationship groups" with an art analysis technique called Visual Thinking Strategies (VTS), which facilitates the identification and examination of various perspectives and emotions elicited by visual art.

Resident physicians, licensed physicians, and advanced practice clinicians across specialties are invited to participate in six evening sessions at the Bechtler Museum of Modern Art. Sessions begin with exploration and group discussion of modern artwork, led by a trained VTS facilitator. The VTS session is followed by an intersession for reflection about the participants' own emotional reactions to the art, their personal well-being, and clinical experiences. Subsequently, trained Balint facilitators lead participants in a Balint session, in which the group explores emotions and perceptions within a patient-physician relationship. The case presented typically bears heavily on the artwork explored during the VTS session. The ambiguous nature of modern art appears to accelerate the Balint process by priming participants to seek alternative viewpoints and engage in deeper emotional processing. Participants report improved insight, empathy, and ability to reflect in their clinical work as a result of their participation in the Art of Medicine.

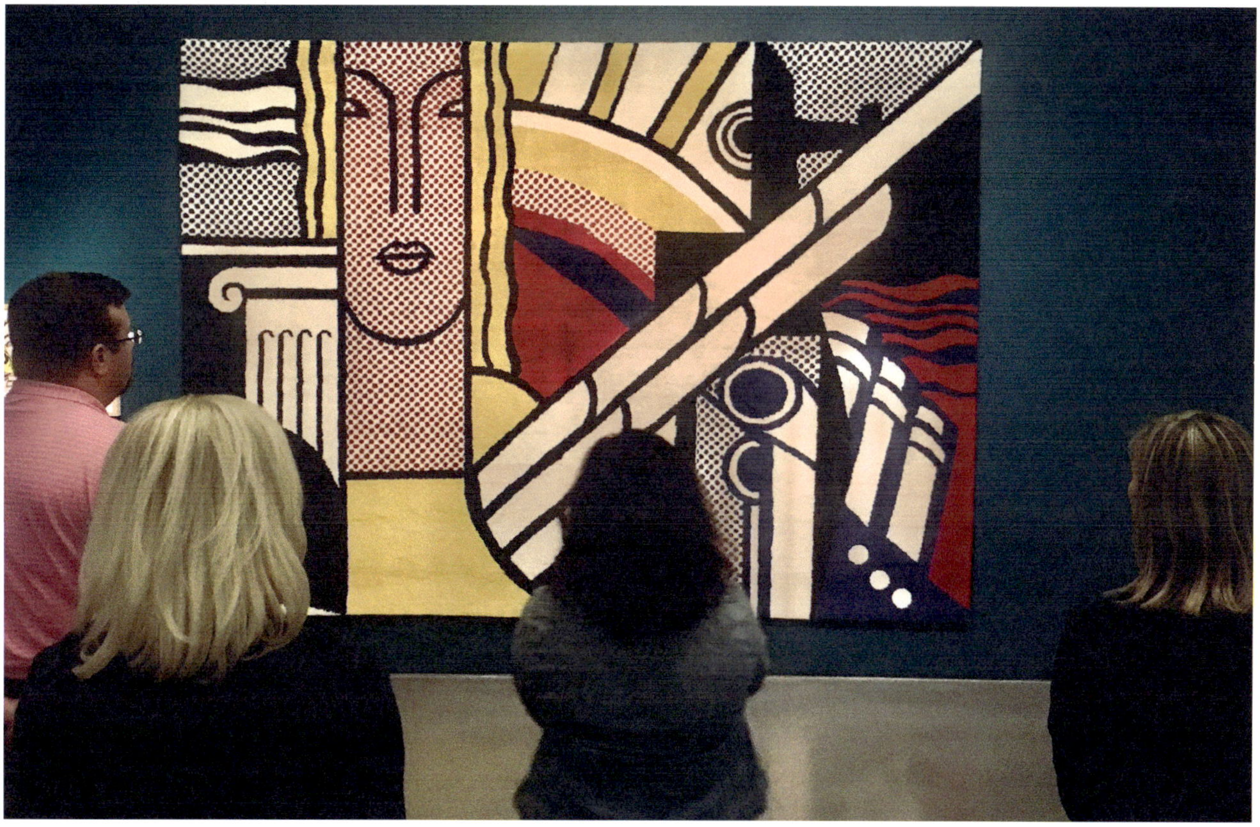

Physicians and advance practice providers examine paintings through the Art of Medicine program at the Bechtler Museum of Modern Art. Image credits: Roy Lichtenstein, Modern Tapestry, *1968, wool and cotton, © Estate of Roy Lichtenstein, Bechtler Museum of Modern Art, Charlotte, North Carolina, USA. Photo © Allison K. Bickett, PhD.*

6. Recommendations for Integrative Approaches

Integrating the arts and humanities into medical education contributes to meeting the diverse learning needs of current and future physicians. Despite great interest and activity around this integration, the evidence that directly links arts and humanities integration with medical education learning outcomes is limited. Indeed, causality is difficult to prove for most educational activities designed to support the complex process of learning to be a physician. More work is needed, and much is underway, to develop theoretical models and robust research and evaluation methods to advance this field. Existing experience, research, and evaluation findings, as well as the great promise of integrative arts and humanities curricula, lead us to believe we should not wait for more rigorous findings to embark on enhanced curriculum development, methods of assessment, and faculty development.

Teams that have cognitive and identity diversity bring many advantages — including increased creativity and problem solving. Partnerships with a variety of individuals who bring unique talents, expertise, and perspectives may ultimately produce learning experiences that are more engaging, robust, and impactful than experiences championed by a passionate individual or small group.[84] Patients, learners, artists, humanities experts, and education and other social science scholars are encouraged to collaborate to optimize creativity and rigor.

Our process of discovery, beginning with a thought leader forum, led to the commissioning of a scoping review and the work of the FRAHME Integration Committee (see Appendix A) and, in turn, to the following broad recommendations for the integration of the arts and humanities into medical education and continuing professional development.

1. Assert that the practice of medicine is an art and a science, requiring a grounding in humanistic values, principles, and skills, including a deep understanding of the human condition.
2. Create more effective arts and humanities integrative models for competency-based teaching and learning in medicine.
3. Enhance the research and evaluation of courses and programs that integrate the arts and humanities into medical education and continuing professional development. These research and evaluation efforts should include measuring learner outcomes beyond satisfaction with the course or program and should follow sound scholarly practices.
4. Design approaches to enhancing trainee and physician well-being that integrate the arts and humanities into medicine.
5. Increase collaboration among scholars of higher education, medical professionals, arts organizations, creative arts therapists, artists, humanities scholars, learners, and patients.
6. Provide professional development offerings that enhance faculties' capacity to design curricula and facilitate the use of models that integrate the arts, humanities, and medicine in training.
7. Investigate effective integrative pedagogical practices and recognize an expansive view of scholarship in academic promotion and tenure processes.

Conclusions

As North American medical education and health care systems continue to rapidly evolve, integrative arts and humanities curricula provide important opportunities for equipping physicians with core competencies for complex 21st-century practice. This report provides an overview of the diverse approaches to such curricula and guidance on their expansion, evaluation, and integration into schools and programs across premedical, undergraduate, graduate, and continuing medical education levels. The FRAHME initiative's commissioned Scoping Review Team developed an emerging theory of practice, the Prism Model.[54] This new model presents four functions of the arts and humanities in medical education derived from qualitative analysis of the published literature: mastering skills, perspective-taking, personal insight, and social advocacy. This model can be a guiding framework for educators that accounts for the complexities inherent to teaching and learning medicine.

Our work to date has revealed rich and diverse educational contributions, and some challenges, of weaving arts and humanities into medical education. Educators should consider several factors when designing curricula, assessing outcomes, and evaluating programs, including challenging assumptions and bringing an open and curious mind to the work, supporting deliberate integration and pedagogy, and mitigating reductionism in approach and assessment. Whether you are a medical educator, clinician, or trainee, we hope this report gives you insights into future practice and opportunities to discuss the complexities of learning the art of medicine.

Appendix A. FRAHME Methods and Strategy

The AAMC began its journey into the role of the arts and humanities in medical education at a thought leaders forum held July 11-12, 2017, in Washington, D.C., with support from the National Endowment for the Humanities (NEH). Forum attendees included medical educators, trainees, and professionals from the arts and humanities. The goals met by that convening were to better understand the current landscape of arts and humanities in medicine and to consider how best to approach a broader effort, including a third monograph in the Foundations series. The activities for the subsequent phases of this initiative were informed by the outcomes of that forum.

In March 2019, the AAMC commissioned and funded a scoping review, detailed in Section 4 of this report. It provides a comprehensive picture of the literature while making judgments about their relevance to the following broadly based research question: *How and why are the arts and humanities being used to educate physicians and interprofessional learners across the developmental spectrum?* The team chosen to conduct the review was from the University of Western Ontario, Penn State College of Medicine, and Mount Saint Vincent University. Led by Lorelei Lingard, PhD (University of Western Ontario), Tracy Moniz, PhD (Mount Saint Vincent University), Maryam Golafshani (University of Western Ontario), and Paul Haidet, MD, MPH (Penn State College of Medicine), the team has a strong track record of scholarship in this domain. The scoping review builds on the team's previous literature reviews, critical analyses, and conceptual frameworks. Section 4 also includes an overview of select scoping review findings — an array of approaches to integrating arts and humanities into medical education.

Beginning in September 2019, the AAMC serially convened a group of educators, clinicians, researchers, historians, humanities scholars, artists, and communication experts from representative member and affiliate institutions around the United States, known as the Arts and Humanities Integration Committee (IC) (see Appendix B for members). Representatives from the Scoping Review Team also participated. The group's charge was to:

- Advise on the overall initiative.
- Articulate the critical arts and humanities foundations for the education of future physicians.
- Recommend the integration of arts and humanities into the professional development of physicians, particularly in the areas of clinical skills and empathic patient-centered care, resilience, communication, tolerance for ambiguity, and other areas as identified through the scoping review process.
- Propose strategies for achieving the recommended need to integrate arts and humanities across the educational and professional development experience of students pursuing the MD degree and physician faculty in practice.
- Consider how to state this recommendation and the consequences to AAMC-member institutions of stating it.
- Serve as or recommend faculty for the new faculty development program to advance the design and evaluation of arts and humanities integration in medical education.

With the support of the NEH, the AAMC is also creating a digital guidebook and a faculty development program for medical educators new to thinking about using arts and humanities in their teaching and those who need further training to evaluate various approaches and develop curricula. A small grants program will provide faculty with funding to pursue educational scholarship that advances research and evaluation of existing integrative arts and humanities curricula. The AAMC is also launching new FRAHME projects to support the creation and sharing of stories and creative works by its constituents. These efforts will include providing outlets to explore and honor health care professionals' experiences during uncertain times.

Appendix B. FRAHME Roster

Arts and Humanities Integration Committee

Laurie Baefsky, DMA
Associate Dean of Research and Strategic Partnerships
College of Arts and Media
University of Colorado Denver

Joanne Braxton, PhD, MDiv
Chief Executive Officer and President
The Braxton Institute for Sustainability, Resiliency and Joy
Adjunct Professor, Family and Community Medicine
Eastern Virginia Medical School

Carlyle H. Chan, MD
Professor of Psychiatry and the Institute for Health and Equity
(Bioethics and Medical Humanities)
Medical College of Wisconsin

Rita Charon, MD, PhD
Professor of Medicine and Medical Humanities and Ethics
Columbia University Vagelos College of Physicians and Surgeons

Issa Lara Combs, MS
Director of Finance and Administration
Chance Academy

Horace DeLisser, MD
Associate for Dean for Diversity and Inclusion
Perelman School of Medicine at the University of Pennsylvania

Quentin Eichbaum, MD, PhD, MPH, MFA
Professor of Medical Education and Administration
Professor of Pathology, Microbiology, and Immunology
Vanderbilt University Medical Center

Cheryl Woods Giscombe, PhD, PMHNP, FAAN
LeVine Distinguished Associate Professor of Quality of Life, Health Promotion, and Wellness
University of North Carolina at Chapel Hill School of Nursing

Deepu Gowda, MD, MPH
Assistant Dean for Medical Education, Associate Professor
Kaiser Permanente School of Medicine

Jeremy Greene, MA, MD, PhD
William H. Welch Professor of Medicine and the History of Medicine
Director, Institute of the History of Medicine
Johns Hopkins University

Therese Jones, PhD
Associate Director of the Center for Bioethics and Humanities
Director of the Arts and Humanities in Healthcare Program
University of Colorado School of Medicine at the Anschutz Medical Campus

Evonne Kaplan-Liss, MD, MPH
Assistant Dean of Narrative Reflection and Patient Communication
TCU and UNTHSC School of Medicine

Catherine Kuhn, MD
Professor of Anesthesiology
Duke University Medical School

Julia Langley
Faculty Director
Georgetown Lombardi Arts and Humanities Program

Jerry Lazarus, MD
Professor of Dermatology
Duke University School of Medicine
National Trust for the Humanities

Daniel Marchalik, MD
Medical Director for Physician Well-being
MedStar Health
Director of the Literature and Medicine Track
Georgetown University School of Medicine

Maren Monsen, MD
Director of the Program in Bioethics and Film
Stanford University

Justin Mutter, MD
Assistant Professor
UVA Center for Health Humanities and Ethics
University of Virginia

Johanna Rian, PhD
Program Director
Dolores Jean Lavins Center for Humanities in Medicine
Mayo Clinic

Robert Rock, MD
Family Medicine Resident
Montefiore Health System

Pamela Schaff, MD, PhD
Associate Professor of Medical Education, Family Medicine, and Pediatrics
Director, Humanities, Ethics/Economics, Art, and the Law (HEAL) Program
Keck School of Medicine of the University of Southern California

Vidya Viswanathan, MD
Founder, Doctors Who Create
Pediatrics Resident
Children's Hospital of Philadelphia

Colleen Wallace, MD
Associate Professor of Pediatrics, Hospitalist Medicine
Program for Humanities in Medicine
Washington University School of Medicine in St. Louis

Katie Watson, JD
Associate Professor of Medical Social Sciences, Medical Education, and Obstetrics and Gynecology
Northwestern University Feinberg School of Medicine

Ray Williams, MA, EdM
Director of Education and Academic Affairs
Blanton Museum of Art
University of Texas at Austin

Association Advisors

Sunil Iyengar, MA
Research and Analysis Director
National Endowment for the Arts

Tom Rudin
Director of the Board on Higher Education and Workforce
Director of the Committee on Women in Science, Engineering, and Medicine
National Academy of Sciences

Victoria Sams, PhD
Program Officer, Division of Education
National Endowment for the Humanities

Scoping Review Team

Tracy Moniz, MA, PhD
Associate Professor, Department of Communication Studies
Mount Saint Vincent University
Adjunct Professor, Department of Pediatrics, Faculty of Medicine
Dalhousie University

Maryam Golafshani, MA
Medical Student
University of Toronto

Carolyn M. Gaspar, MSc
PhD student, Faculty of Health
Dalhousie University

Nancy E. Adams, MLIS, EdD
Associate Librarian and Assistant Dean of Foundational Sciences
Penn State College of Medicine

Paul Haidet, MD, MPH
Director of Medical Education Research
Woodward Center for Excellence in Health Sciences Education
Penn State College of Medicine.

Javeed Sukhera, MD, PhD
Associate Professor
Departments of Psychiatry/Pediatrics
Scientist, Centre for Education Research and Innovation
Schulich School of Medicine and Dentistry, Western University

Rebecca L. Volpe, PhD
Assistant Professor and Vice Chair for Education
Department of Humanities, Penn State College of Medicine
Director of the Clinical Ethics Consultation Service
Milton S. Hershey Medical Center

Claire de Boer, MS
Director of the Doctors Kienle Center for Humanistic Medicine
Founding Director of Center Stage Arts in Health
Penn State College of Medicine and Penn State Health
Milton S. Hershey Medical Center
President of the National Organization for Arts in Health

Lorelei Lingard, MA, PhD
Professor, Department of Medicine
Scientist, Centre for Education Research and Innovation
Schulich School of Medicine and Dentistry, Western University

AAMC Core Project Team

Virginia Bush, PMP
Project Manager
Strategic Initiatives and Partnerships in Medical Education

Elizabeth Gaufberg, MD, MPH
Senior Consultant, AAMC
Associate Professor of Medicine and Psychiatry, Harvard Medical School
Director, Center for Professional and Academic Development, The Cambridge Health Alliance

Lisa Howley, PhD, MEd
Senior Director, Strategic Initiatives and Partnerships in Medical Education, AAMC
Adjunct Associate Professor, UNC School of Medicine

Brandy King, MLIS
Senior Consultant, AAMC
Librarian
Knowledge Linking

Mallory Lee, MA
Administrative Support Specialist
Strategic Initiatives and Partnerships in Medical Education

Beatrice Schmider, MA
Executive Assistant II
Office of Medical Education

Alison Whelan, MD
Chief Medical Education Officer

AAMC Supporting Staff

Amy Addams
Director, Student Affairs Alignment and Holistic Review

Deric Corlew, PhD
Director, Business Development

Jennifer Faerberg, MHSA
Director, Advancing Clinical Leadership and Quality

Anne Farmakidis, MPS
Senior Director, Educational Resources and Scholarship

Toni Gallo, MA
Senior Staff Editor, *Academic Medicine*
Lead, Education Resources and Scholarship

John Nash
Operations Manager
Education Resources and Scholarship

AAMC

References

1. AAMC, Howard Hughes Medical Institute. *The Scientific Foundations for Future Physicians.* Washington, DC: AAMC; 2009. https://www.aamc.org/system/files?file=2020-02/scientificfoundationsforfuturephysicians.pdf.

2. AAMC. *Behavioral and Social Science Foundations for Future Physicians.* Washington, DC: AAMC; 2011. https://www.aamc.org/system/files/d/1/271020-behavioralandsocialsciencefoundationsforfuturephysicians.pdf.

3. National Endowment for the Humanities. What are the humanities? https://www.neh.gov/about. Accessed May 1, 2020.

4. National Academies of Sciences, Engineering, and Medicine. *The Integration of the Humanities and Arts With Sciences, Engineering, and Medicine in Higher Education: Branches From the Same Tree.* Washington, DC: National Academies Press; 2018. doi:https://doi.org/10.17226/24988.

5. Kulasegaram KM, Martimianakis MA, Mylopoulos M, Whitehead CR, Woods NN. Cognition before curriculum: rethinking the integration of basic science and clinical learning. *Acad Med.* 2013;88(10):1578-1585. doi:10.1097/ACM.0b013e3182a45def.

6. Muller JH, Jain S, Loeser H, Irby DM. Lessons learned about integrating a medical school curriculum: perceptions of students, faculty and curriculum leaders. *Med Educ.* 2008;42(8):778-785. doi:10.1111/j.1365-2923.2008.03110.x.

7. Quintero GA, Vergel J, Arredondo M, Ariza MC, Gómez P, Pinzon-Barrios AM. Integrated medical curriculum: advantages and disadvantages. *J Med Educ Curric Dev.* 2016;3:133-137. doi:10.4137/jmecd.S18920.

8. Brauer DG, Ferguson KJ. The integrated curriculum in medical education: AMEE Guide No. 96. *Med Teach.* 2015;37(4):312-322. doi:10.3109/0142159x.2014.970998.

9. Cyr PR, Schirmer JM, Hayes V, Martineau C, Keane M. Integrating interprofessional case scenarios, allied embedded actors, and teaching into formative observed structured clinical exams. *Fam Med.* 2020;52(3):209-212. doi:10.22454/FamMed.2020.760357.

10. Peiris-John R, Selak V, Robb G, et al. The state of quality improvement teaching in medical schools: a systematic review. *J Surg Educ.* 2020;77(4):889-904. doi:10.1016/j.jsurg.2020.01.003.

11. Green AR, Betancourt JR, Park ER, Greer JA, Donahue EJ, Weissman JS. Providing culturally competent care: residents in HRSA Title VII funded residency programs feel better prepared. *Acad Med.* 2008;83(11):1071-1079. doi:10.1097/ACM.0b013e3181890b16.

12. Charon R. *Narrative Medicine: Honoring the Stories of Illness.* New York, NY: Oxford University Press; 2006.

13. Mangione S, Chakraborti C, Staltari G, et al. Medical students' exposure to the humanities correlates with positive personal qualities and reduced burnout: a multi-institutional U.S. survey. *J Gen Intern Med.* 2018;33(5):628-634. doi:10.1007/s11606-017-4275-8.

14. Wald HS, White J, Reis SP, Esquibel AY, Anthony D. Grappling with complexity: medical students' reflective writings about challenging patient encounters as a window into professional identity formation. *Med Teach.* 2019;41(2):152-160. doi:10.1080/0142159x.2018.1475727.

15. Marchalik D, Jurecic A. Novel remedies. *Lancet.* 2015;386(10000):1223. doi:10.1016/s0140-6736(15)00301-3.

16. National Library of Medicine. Greek medicine. 2002; http://www.nlm.nih.gov/hmd/greek/greek_oath.html. Accessed May 24, 2020.

17. Flexner A. *Medical Education in the United Sates and Canada.* New York, NY: Carnegie Foundation for the Advancement of Teaching; 1910.

18. Osler W. The reserves of life. *St Mary's Hospital Gazette.* 1907;13:95-98.

19. Snow CP. Two cultures. *Science.* 1959;130(3373):419. doi:10.1126/science.130.3373.419.

20. Kollmer Horton ME. The orphan child: humanities in modern medical education. *Philos Ethics Humanit Med.* 2019;14(1):1. doi:10.1186/s13010-018-0067-y.

21. Charon R. The patient-physician relationship. Narrative medicine: a model for empathy, reflection, profession, and trust. *JAMA.* 2001;286(15):1897-1902. doi:10.1001/jama.286.15.1897.

22. Charon R. The shock of attention. *Enthymema.* 2016;16:6-17. doi:https://doi.org/10.13130/2037-2426/7437.

23. DasGupta S. Narrative humility. *Lancet.* 2008;371(9617):980-981. doi:10.1016/s0140-6736(08)60440-7.

24. Evans HM, Greaves DA. Ten years of medical humanities: a decade in the life of a journal and a discipline. *Med Humanit.* 2010;36(2):66-68. doi:10.1136/jmh.2010.005603.

25. Doukas DJ, McCullough LB, Wear S. Medical education in medical ethics and humanities as the foundation for developing medical professionalism. Perspective. *Acad Med.* 2012;87(3):334-341. doi:10.1097/ACM.0b013e318244728c.

26. Doukas DJ, McCullough LB, Wear S, et al. The challenge of promoting professionalism through medical ethics and humanities education. *Acad Med.* 2013;88(11):1624-1629. doi:10.1097/ACM.0b013e3182a7f8e3.

27. Health Humanities Consortium. About the Health Humanities Consortium. https://healthhumanitiesconsortium.com/about/. Accessed May 22, 2020.

28. Pitman B. *The Art of Examination: Art Museum and Medical School Partnerships — Forum Report.* Dallas, TX: The University of Texas at Dallas; October 2016.

29. AAMC. Content documentation in required courses and elective courses. https://www.aamc.org/initiatives/cir/406462/06a.html. Accessed May 22, 2020.

30. Liaison Committee on Medical Education. *Functions and Structure of a Medical School: Standards for Accreditation of Medical Education Programs Leading to the MD Degree.* March 2020. https://lcme.org/wp-content/uploads/filebase/standards/2021-22_Functions-and-Structure_2020-03-31.docx.

31. Lamb E, Berry S, Jones T. *Health Humanities Baccalaureate Programs in the United States.* Cleveland, OH: Case Western Reserve University School of Medicine; 2020.

32. Jones T, Blackie M, Garden R, Wear D. The almost right word: the move from medical to health humanities. *Acad Med.* 2017;92(7):932-935. doi:10.1097/acm.0000000000001518.

33. Kumagai AK, Wear D. "Making strange": a role for the humanities in medical education. *Acad Med.* 2014;89(7):973-977. doi:10.1097/acm.0000000000000269.

34. Green MJ. Comics and medicine: peering into the process of professional identity formation. *Acad Med.* 2015;90(6):774-779. doi:10.1097/acm.0000000000000703.

35. Reis SP, Wald HS. Contemplating medicine during the Third Reich: scaffolding professional identity formation for medical students. *Acad Med.* 2015;90(6):770-773. doi:10.1097/acm.0000000000000716.

36. Shapiro J, Nixon LL, Wear SE, Doukas DJ. Medical professionalism: what the study of literature can contribute to the conversation. *Philos Ethics Humanit Med.* 2015;10:10. doi:10.1186/s13010-015-0030-0.

37. Shapiro J, Youm J, Heare M, et al. Medical students' efforts to integrate and/or reclaim authentic identity: insights from a mask-making exercise. *J Med Humanit.* 2018;39(4):483-501. doi:10.1007/s10912-018-9534-0.

38. Miller E, Balmer D, Hermann N, Graham G, Charon R. Sounding narrative medicine: studying students' professional identity development at Columbia University College of Physicians and Surgeons. *Acad Med.* 2014;89(2):335-342. doi:10.1097/acm.0000000000000098.

39. Shapiro J, Coulehan J, Wear D, Montello M. Medical humanities and their discontents: definitions, critiques, and implications. *Acad Med.* 2009;84(2):192-198. doi:10.1097/ACM.0b013e3181938bca.

40. Frank AW. Asking the right question about pain: narrative and phronesis. *Lit Med.* 2004;23(2):209-225. doi:10.1353/lm.2005.0003.

41. Schwartz B, Sharpe K. *Practical Wisdom: The Right Way To Do the Right Thing.* New York, NY: Riverhead Books; 2010.

42. Barber JP. Integration of learning: a grounded theory analysis of college students' learning. *Am Edu Res J.* 2012;49(3):590-617. doi:https://doi.org/10.3102/0002831212437854.

43. Wellbery C, McAteer RA. The art of observation: a pedagogical framework. *Acad Med.* 2015;90(12):1624-1630. doi:10.1097/acm.0000000000000801.

44. Doctors Who Create. https://www.doctorswhocreate.com/. Accessed June 19, 2020.

45. Los Angeles Doctors Symphony Orchestra. https://ladso.org/. Accessed June 19, 2020.

46. Browne K. Why Doctors Write: Finding Humanity in Medicine. Documentary film in production. Preview available at https://vimeo.com/137260974.

47. Walsh C. Taking a break for beauty. *Harvard Gazette* 2020;May 27. https://news.harvard.edu/gazette/story/2020/05/art-museums-uses-collections-to-help-doctors-decompress/. Accessed May 27, 2020.

48. Fogarty CT. Fifty-five word stories: "small jewels" for personal reflection and teaching. *Fam Med.* 2010;42(6):400-402. doi:10.7205/MILMED-D-16-00195.

49. Roberts TJ, Ringler T, Krahn D, Ahearn E. The My Life, My Story program: sustained impact of veterans' personal narratives on healthcare providers 5 years after implementation. *Health Commun.* 2020:1-8. doi:10.1080/10410236.2020.1719316.

50. Watson K. Serious play: teaching medical skills with improvisational theater techniques. Perspective. *Acad Med.* 2011;86(10):1260-1265. doi:10.1097/ACM.0b013e31822cf858.

51. Marchalik D. The return to literature-making doctors matter in the new era of medicine. *Acad Med.* 2017;92(12):1665-1667. doi:10.1097/acm.0000000000001986.

52. Batalden P, Leach D, Swing S, Dreyfus H, Dreyfus S. General competencies and accreditation in graduate medical education. *Health Aff (Millwood).* 2002;21(5):103-111. doi:10.1377/hlthaff.21.5.103.

53. Fins JJ, Pohl B, Doukas DJ. In praise of the humanities in academic medicine. Values, metrics, and ethics in uncertain times. *Camb Q Healthc Ethics.* 2013;22(4):355-364. doi:10.1017/s0963180113000200.

54. Moniz T, Golafshani M, Gaspar C, et al. Prism Model for Integrating Arts and Humanities into Medical Education. *Acad Med.* In press.

55. Dennhardt S, Apramian T, Lingard L, Torabi N, Arntfield S. Rethinking research in the medical humanities: a scoping review and narrative synthesis of quantitative outcome studies. *Med Educ.* 2016;50(3):285-299. doi:10.1111/medu.12812.

56. Gawande A. Cowboys and pit crews. *The New Yorker* 2011;May 26. http://www.newyorker.com/news/news-desk/cowboys-and-pit-crews.

57. Klugman CM, Peel J, Beckmann-Mendez D. Art rounds: teaching interprofessional students visual thinking strategies at one school. *Acad Med.* 2011;86(10):1266-1271. doi:10.1097/ACM.0b013e31822c1427.

58. Katz JT, Khoshbin S. Can visual arts training improve physician performance? *Trans Am Clin Climatol Assoc.* 2014;125:331-342.

59. Zelenski AB, Saldivar N, Park LS, Schoenleber V, Osman F, Kraemer S. Interprofessional improv: using theater techniques to teach health professions students empathy in teams. *Acad Med.* 2020. Published ahead of print. doi:10.1097/acm.0000000000003420.

60. Ariely D, Lanier WL. Disturbing trends in physician burnout and satisfaction with work-life balance: dealing with malady among the nation's healers. *Mayo Clin Proc.* 2015;90(12):1593-1596. doi:10.1016/j.mayocp.2015.10.004.

61. Litz BT, Stein N, Delaney E, et al. Moral injury and moral repair in war veterans: a preliminary model and intervention strategy. *Clin Psychol Rev.* 2009;29(8):695-706. doi:10.1016/j.cpr.2009.07.003.

62. Bentwich ME, Gilbey P. More than visual literacy: art and the enhancement of tolerance for ambiguity and empathy. *BMC Med Educ.* 2017;17(1):200. doi:10.1186/s12909-017-1028-7.

63. Shapiro J, Rucker L, Robitshek D. Teaching the art of doctoring: an innovative medical student elective. *Med Teach.* 2006;28(1):30-35. doi:10.1080/01421590600568348.

64. Standford WellMD Center. Projects and partners. https://wellmd.stanford.edu/center1/projects.html. Accessed June 16, 2020.

65. Flock E. Burnout is rampant among doctors and nurses. Can the arts help? *PBS NewsHour.* 2019. https://www.pbs.org/newshour/arts/burnout-is-rampant-among-doctors-and-nurses-can-the-arts-help. Accessed May 24, 2020.

66. Braxton Institute. Transforming Moral Injury Across the Professions: Cultivating Moral Resilience Through Reflective Writing and Contemplative Practice. https://www.braxtoninstitute.org/human-ecology-of-racism-1/2019/5/29/transforming-moral-injury-across-the-professions. Accessed May 26, 2020.

67. Jones T. Moving pictures: visual culture/visual activism in the health humanities classroom. In: Banner O, Carlin N, Cole T, eds. *Teaching Health Humanities*. New York, NY: Oxford University Press; 2019.

68. Wear D, Kumagai AK, Varley J, Zarconi J. Cultural competency 2.0: exploring the concept of "difference" in engagement with the other. *Acad Med*. 2012;87(6):752-758. doi:10.1097/ACM.0b013e318253cef8.

69. Garden R. Who speaks for whom? Health humanities and the ethics of representation. *Med Humanit*. 2015;41(2):77-80. doi:10.1136/medhum-2014-010642.

70. Bell SK, Etchegaray JM, Gaufberg E, et al. A multi-stakeholder consensus-driven research agenda for better understanding and supporting the emotional impact of harmful events on patients and families. *Jt Comm J Qual Patient Saf*. 2018;44(7):424-435. doi:10.1016/j.jcjq.2018.03.007.

71. Gaufberg E, Olmsted MW, Bell SK. Third things as inspiration and artifact: a multi-stakeholder qualitative approach to understand patient and family emotions after harmful events. *J Med Humanit*. 2019;40(4):489-504. doi:10.1007/s10912-019-09563-z.

72. White A. Xenophobia in the time of quarantines. *Johns Hopkins News and Publications*. 2020;April 10. https://www.hopkinsmedicine.org/news/articles/xenophobia-in-the-time-of-quarantines. Accessed May 24, 2020.

73. Wear D, Zarconi J, Garden R, Jones T. Reflection in/and writing: pedagogy and practice in medical education. *Acad Med*. 2012;87(5):603-609. doi:10.1097/ACM.0b013e31824d22e9.

74. Gooding H, Quinn M, Martin B, Charrow A, Katz J. Fostering humanism in medicine through art and reflection. *JME*. 2016;41(2):123-130. doi:10.1080/10598650.2016.1169732.

75. Naghshineh S, Hafler JP, Miller AR, et al. Formal art observation training improves medical students' visual diagnostic skills. *J Gen Intern Med*. 2008;23(7):991-997. doi:10.1007/s11606-008-0667-0.

76. Kern D, Thomas P, Hughes M. *Curriculum Development for Medical Education: A Six-Step Approach*. 3rd ed. Baltimore, MD: Johns Hopkins University Press; 2016.

77. Haidet P, Jarecke J, Adams NE, et al. A guiding framework to maximise the power of the arts in medical education: a systematic review and metasynthesis. *Med Educ*. 2016;50(3):320-331. doi:10.1111/medu.12925.

78. American Educational Research Association. What is education research? https://www.aera.net/About-AERA/What-is-Education-Research. Accessed May 22, 2020.

79. Patton M. *Utilization-Focused Evaluation: The New Century Text*. 3rd ed. Thousand Oaks, CA: Sage; 1997.

80. Moniz T, Golafshani M, Gaspar C, et al. How are the arts and humanities used in medical education?: Synthesis results of a scoping review of published literature. *Acad Med*. In press.

81. Gowda D, Dubroff R, Willieme A, Swan-Sein A, Capello C. Art as sanctuary: a four-year mixed-methods evaluation of a visual art course addressing uncertainty through reflection. *Acad Med*. 2018;93(11S AAMC Learn Serve Lead: Proceedings of the 57th Annual Research in Medical Education Sessions):S8-S13. doi:10.1097/acm.0000000000002379.

82. Boyer EL. *Scholarship Reconsidered: Priorities of the Professoriate*. Princeton, NJ: Carnegie Foundation for the Advancement of Teaching;1990.

83. Eichbaum QG. Thinking about thinking and emotion: the metacognitive approach to the medical humanities that integrates the humanities with the basic and clinical sciences. *Perm J*. 2014;18(4):64-75. doi:10.7812/tpp/14-027.

84. Hong L, Page SE. Groups of diverse problem solvers can outperform groups of high-ability problem solvers. *Proc Natl Acad Sci USA*. 2004;101(46):16385-16389. doi:10.1073/pnas.0403723101.